Quick Start for Correctional Nurses

Is Correctional Nursing for You?

Other books by Lorry Schoenly

*The Wizard of Oz Guide
to Correctional Nursing*

*Correctional Health Care
Patient Safety Handbook*

The Correctional Nurse Manifesto

Essentials of Correctional Nursing

Quick Start for Correctional Nurses

Is Correctional Nursing for You?

Lorry Schoenly, PhD, RN, CCHP-RN
Correctional Health Care Consultant

Enchanted Mountain Press

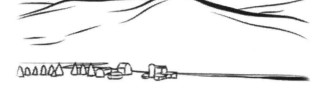

Quick Start for Correctional Nurses
Is Correctional Nursing for You?

Copyright © 2016 Lorry Schoenly

CorrectionalNurse.Net

Published in the United States by Enchanted Mountain Press

ISBN: 978-0-9912942-9-9

Contents

Introduction to the Quick Start for Correctional Nurses Series

Welcome to the *Quick Start for Correctional Nurses Series* of brief books intended to jumpstart your correctional nursing practice. Each book in the series takes only an hour or two to read and is packed with essential and practical information on a specific topic important to correctional nurses. Some books cover nursing processes like sick call and medication administration while others deal with specific patient populations like female inmates or juveniles. Still others explore issues of concern to correctional nurses such as self-care needs and dealing with inmates.

Besides being packed with information, the Quick Start Series includes additional links and resources found on a special page of the CorrectionalNurse.Net blog. Access an expanding list of documents and links at correctionalnurse.net/quickstart.

Whether you are just discovering the world of correctional nursing, have started your first position in a jail or prison, or been in the field a while, the *Quick Start for Correctional Nurses Series* has something for you.

Why Should You Consider Becoming a Correctional Nurse?

Have you ever thought about working behind bars? For many nurses, providing health care in a jail or prison is not even a consideration when deciding on a career direction. In fact, many practicing in the criminal justice system consider themselves to be 'accidental' correctional nurses. Must nurses have little contact with the criminal justice system in nursing school and so are unlikely to choose the specialty. In fact, the general public would rather not think about our patient population. Prisons are often located in out-of-the-way places and the patient population is invisible to most people. Yet over two million Americans are currently behind bars; that is a lot of people in need of health care. And, as at least 95% of prisoners will eventually be released, correctional health care affects public health in a big way.

It takes a special person to practice nursing. Nurses must jump into the lives of their patients at a rough point. Illness, injury, and suffering can be ugly, intense, and deeply painful. We deal with body fluids, needles, gaping wounds, and heart-wrenching loss and must take it all in stride.

It takes a special nurse to practice correctional nursing. The criminal justice system is an unlikely health care environment and prisoners are a unique patient population. Here, illness, injury, and

3

suffering are treated in the midst of heightened security, reduced resources, and isolation.

Yet many nurses find their calling in this unusual health care setting. The variety and nature of patient health needs and the opportunity to bring care and concern into a dehumanizing situation can be unexpected job satisfiers. Correctional nurses deal with a population of disadvantaged and vulnerable patients in a difficult time of life. Lack of prior health care contact means nurses can care for patients with unusual conditions along with the mundane ones. Correctional nursing has been described as 'real' nursing as incarcerated patients need health teaching, self-care skills, and chronic disease management. Correctional nursing practice is autonomous and self-directed.

Is correctional nursing for you? Find out in the pages of this short book. Take a few hours to explore the many facets of correctional nursing practice. Look behind the curtain into this hidden practice setting. Discover this well-kept nursing secret and decide if you should consider becoming a correctional nurse. Over two million incarcerated patients need you!

What Makes Correctional Nursing a Satisfying Career Choice?

Talk to correctional nurses for very long and you will come across stories of encountering disrespect and downright disbelief from among their nurse colleagues in more traditional health care settings.

It is not uncommon to hear from other nurses "Why would you work THERE?" "Can't you get a REAL nurse job?" "Aren't you ruining your career?" Yes, many nurses consider working in a jail or prison as a choice of desperation rather than desire. It may be surprising for these nurses to hear from correctional nurses that working in a jail or prison was a satisfying career choice.

Although research on the correctional nurse role is minimal, a few have evaluated the unique nature of correctional nursing practice and revealed professional job satisfiers. For example, Flanagan and Flanagan in 2001 looked into correctional nursing practice and found that patient teaching, counseling, and physical assessment were primary components of the role. Maroney in 2005 surveyed nurses working in New York state prisons and found that independent and autonomous practice were job satisfiers. Autonomous practice also emerged as a theme in nurse responses to the research survey. Here are concepts that emerge when talking with long-time correctional nurses about what keeps them in the specialty.

Autonomy

Correctional nurses are most often the primary care provider in a correctional setting. Medical staff are likely to have limited hours onsite and then be available on-call. Nurses are the first care provider to evaluate patient concerns and then determine care provision or access to advanced providers such as physicians or dentists. Nursing sick call, in particular, is an exceedingly autonomous practice as nurses evaluate patient symptoms and determine and deliver treatment based on medically-approved protocols.

Assessment

The autonomous nature of correctional nursing practice requires excellent assessment skills and the accompanying clinical judgment to make sense of the assessment findings. Physical assessment and symptom evaluation must be thorough and accurate in order to be conveyed and acted upon by medical and mental health providers, when necessary.

Patient Teaching

Incarcerated patients are less likely to be informed about their health status and often enter the correctional setting with untreated conditions. Health assessments can reveal new diseases such as diabetes or hypertension that require development of self-management habits. This leads to a great need for patient teaching. The high rates of learning disabilities and poor reading skills among the inmate patient population require patience and creative teaching strategies.

Scope of Practice

Correctional nurses, especially those working in small medical units, make use of their full scope of practice in providing nursing care. The variety of conditions, many unusual in traditional settings, and the need to provide as much health care as possible within the facility, maximize nursing care practice. Few other nursing roles allow for a nurse to practice to the full scope of licensure.

Change the Conversation Dynamic

If you are seeking to enter the correctional nursing specialty, be prepared for surprised responses from your nurse colleagues. They are likely to lack understanding about the specialty or the satisfying aspects of working behind bars. For any of us in correctional health care, it can be easy to share the downside of our specialty. Who doesn't have a story to share about a manipulative patient or a hair-raising emergency in the tiers? However, sharing your job satisfaction stories about calming a young and anxious first-time inmate during health screening, teaching a newly discovered diabetic, or solving the puzzle of a strange headache may just overcome skepticism and recruit a new nurse to our specialty. Check out the Appendix in this book for some meaningful stories about correctional nursing practice.

Six Signs You Were Destined to Be a Correctional Nurse

Most nurses work in jails and prisons by accident. The invisible world of correctional nursing is discovered through a job notice, a friend, or by necessity when other nursing jobs were scarce.

You will not meet a correctional nurse who wanted to be one from childhood or remembers a parent's comment, "I hope you grow up to be a jail nurse". Yet, you may have been destined to be a correctional nurse. Here are six signs that indicate your stars were aligning and steering you into a correctional nursing career, even at a young age.

You Can Stand Your Ground with Bullies

Did you naturally stand up to bullies and find timid friends seeking out your protection when they couldn't fend for themselves? Have you always had a determination to seek out justice in an unfair situation or root for the underdog when watching movies? These are signs that you were destined to be a correctional nurse.

Correctional nurses often find themselves in challenging ethical situations where standing up for what is just and right may be required. Brutality is, unfortunately, common in some correctional practice settings. Correctional nurses may need to speak out about unethical practices they see; and they may need to do it without much administrative support. This can require unshakable core beliefs and values while being tolerant of the beliefs and values of others, including patients and officers.

You are Good at Getting People to Confess

Did you always know when something was up with a sibling or child? Were you always able to get that secret out of a friend? This is a good sign that you were destined to be a correctional nurse.

Correctional patients usually have something to hide; whether drug use, alcohol consumption, or suicide contemplation. Nurses able to quickly obtain truthful responses to questions about social, psychological, and medical histories do well in this field.

No One Can Pull One Over On You

Were you the one who always figured out the surprise birthday party or called a school mate out on trying to get you to give them your algebra homework? This is another good sign that you were destined to be a correctional nurse. Plenty of our patients look for ways to manipulate or con staff members into doing their bidding. Correctional nurses need to remain objectively caring while always being alert for the con.

Foul Language and Dirty Words Don't Bother You

Have you always been able to withstand a barrage of blue language in the school yard or locker room? Maybe you were even one of the foul language gabbers! In any case, this is a sign you were destined to be a correctional nurse.

Although there are exceptions, plenty of our patients talk dirty and pepper their conversations with 4-letter words. Some entertain themselves by using foul language to surprise or shock. Others swear to bully or manipulate. In any case, being able to listen past the language and address the real issue is a successful correctional nursing practice.

You Don't Embarrass Easily and Nothing Surprises You

When you were growing up, were friends able to share embarrassing information without worry that you would judge them? Did you build up a tolerance for bathroom humor and bodily fluids in interacting with your siblings? This all contributed to your destiny as a correctional nurse.

Not only must correctional nurses have a tolerance for foul language, but some settings also provide surprising visual and tactile experiences during the work day. Some patients are prone to act out by exposing body parts or tossing bodily fluids. Nursing rounds in behavioral segregation units can be embarrassing and anxiety-producing for some nurses. A matter-of-fact no-nonsense attitude toward socially unacceptable behavior will rule the day.

You Have Always Been Able to Balance Your Life

Have you always been able to balance the craziness of life with your own sense of purpose and direction? Were you the rock of sensibility that friends turned to when their world was coming apart? This is an excellent sign that you were destined to become a correctional nurse.

Working in a correctional setting can be stressful. Correctional nurses regularly hear patient stories of abuse and trauma. We may see harsh treatment among inmates and staff. As healers and caregivers, we are prone to take on the burdens of our patients; sometimes without even being aware of it. Effective nursing in the criminal justice system requires that we are fully there for our patients while keeping balance in our own lives when we leave the workplace.

Five Personality Traits of a Correctional Nurse

Personality traits can also affect satisfaction in correctional nursing practice. Although more research is needed, there is some indication that nurses are drawn to a particular specialty based on personality traits.

Psychologists have been studying human personality for decades and have settled on a model of five key factors to explain various personality characteristics. The theory is that each of us has a combination of these five factors in varying degrees that create our unique personality. A link to a version of the Big Five Personality Test can be found at correctionalnurse.net/quickstart.

How might these personality traits work toward an ideal alignment in correctional nursing practice? Here are some ideas.

Openness

This personality trait involves the appreciation of the new and unusual. It also involves openness to unconventional thoughts or unusual ideas. A nurse with a high level of this personality trait might be less judgmental of a patient's lifestyle choices. Also, an abundance of this trait would allow a nurse to take the risk in trying out a position in a jail or prison.

Correctional nursing is both unconventional and nontraditional as a practice setting. Our patient population often consists of those who have made unpopular lifestyle choices. Correctional nurses must be able to look beyond these characteristics to be able to care for patients in the criminal justice system.

Conscientiousness

Conscientiousness as a personality trait deals with self-regulation and impulse control, as well as a preference for planned rather than spontaneous behavior. Nurses high in this personality trait are orderly and plan ahead.

Correctional nurses deal with a patient population generally low in the conscientiousness trait. Poor impulse control and self-management often land people behind bars. Nurses who provide correctional health care must be able to control their own impulses and help their patients do the same. Correctional nurses must be able to think ahead to potential safety issues and plan accordingly.

Extroversion

The personality trait of extroversion explains a person's connection with the world outside themselves. High extroversion indicates a high connection with the social world, while low extroversion indicates less need for social connection.

Neither high nor low extroversion is necessarily needed for enjoyment of the correctional nurse specialty. This trait in high degree may lead an individual to be drawn in to a 'con', while a nurse scoring lower in this trait may be more likely to internalize trauma and stress leading to vicarious trauma or burnout.

Agreeableness

The agreeableness trait deals with the level of concern for social harmony. Nurses high in this trait are more trusting and willing to compromise their interests in order to get along with others. They are more likely to extend themselves for others. Nurses low in this trait place a higher value on self-interest and are more likely to be skeptical about the motives of others.

A balance in this trait is helpful in correctional nursing practice. High levels of agreeableness can lead to leniency in dealing with inmate manipulation while low levels can lead to cynicism toward inmate concerns. Balanced agreeableness is also helpful when negotiating with custody staff. As health care is not the primary mission of a correctional facility, nurses frequently need to work out an agreeable solution to a patient issue that takes into consideration both security and health care concerns.

Neuroticism

The neuroticism personality trait deals with emotional stability. Nurses who score high in the neuroticism trait are emotionally reactive and sensitive to stress. Even normal situations can appear threatening to those with very high levels of this trait. On the other end of the spectrum, nurses low in this trait regulate emotions and have less negative feelings, managing stress well.

Nurses on the lower end of the neuroticism scale do better in the correctional setting, and in life, in general, for that matter. A calm, even temper is needed to deal daily with this patient population and the stresses of personal security that are a part of correctional practice.

Of course, this application of the big five personality traits to correctional nursing practice is neither scientific nor validated in practice, but comes from experience working with nurses both happy and unhappy in the correctional specialty. Consider your personality traits and how they might affect your nursing practice in a jail or prison.

Jail or Prison
– What's the Diff?

Jails and prisons are not the same. The type of health care services you provide and the patient community is varied - although there are similar components to each. Here is a short comparison of these two types of correctional settings and how the type of facility may affect nursing practice.

Jail

A jail is a correctional facility usually operated by the local city or county government and holds an arrestee awaiting trial and sentencing. Many jails also hold those sentenced for crimes with less than 12 months' time to serve. Thus, a jail will have detained (not put on trial) and sentenced (put on trial and found guilty) inmates who might be housed in different areas of the facility.

The patient community in a jail will include a large percentage withdrawing from a variety of drugs and alcohol. Newly arriving inmates may have acute conditions related to the circumstances of their arrest. Many of those booked into the jail will be released in a mere hours or days. For example, some large urban areas regularly perform 'sweeps' of the neighborhoods, clearing the streets of vagrants and homeless.

Dealing with immediate needs and urgent medical or mental health issues are top priorities in a jail. Patients are less likely to be under consistent medical care and may have untreated infectious diseases, such as tuberculosis or sexually transmitted infections. Rapid turnover in jails means a high possibility of missed diagnoses and incomplete treatment.

For the most part, jails have both male and female inmates.

Prison

A prison, on the other hand, is a correctional facility operated by the state or federal government for those who have been tried and sentenced. Prisons have a range of security levels depending on the type of sentence of the inmate, usually based on degree of potential for violence. Leveling ranges from minimum to medium to maximum security (where death row and highly volatile/violent inmates are housed). By the time an inmate reaches the prison setting, substance detoxification has taken place and acute conditions stabilized. Even with this increased predictability, prison nursing also includes emergency evaluation and treatment.

Prison nursing usually involves management of chronic conditions and ambulatory care. If the prison complex includes work sites such as a farm or metal shop, nurses may be evaluating inmates for ability to be assigned or deferred from various levels of work details. Prisons tend to be located in remote areas away from high population centers and, therefore, can have difficulty recruiting qualified personnel.

Prisons generally have either male or female inmates. Genders are rarely mixed in a prison system.

Which Type of Nursing Would Appeal to You?

Nurses who end up enjoying the jail environment like a fast-paced constantly changing situation. These are usually the same nurses who thrive in an urban emergency room, as there are similarities in the type of conditions encountered. Jail nursing can involve interesting assessment situations and a good bit of trauma evaluation. Major conditions addressed include substance withdrawal, contagious disease, and suicide prevention.

The prison environment has more opportunity for planning and scheduling as the inmate community will be around longer, generating the ability to develop a therapeutic relationship. There is greater involvement in medication management, patient education, and diagnostics. Nurses who value a long-term relationship and the opportunity to improve health outcomes over time tend to prefer prison nursing as a correctional specialty.

Who Employs
Correctional Nurses?

If you are thinking about jumping into the interesting world of correctional nursing, you may be looking for employers in all the wrong places. Unlike a traditional health care setting, correctional health care units may not be managed in-house, although many are. Below is a primer on various correctional health care management structures.

Governmental Agencies (Self-Operated)

Most correctional nurses do work for the same employer as their custody peers. In other words, they are hired by the jail or prison administrators. Currently about 58% of correctional health care facilities are in this category. The industry calls this 'self-operated' or 'self-op'. Health care managers in this management structure are a part of the organizational hierarchy and reporting framework. This can be a great advantage for making changes or obtaining resources as the health care manager is on parity with other services, therefore fostering support for inmate medical needs. There are disadvantages to this arrangement, as well. Although the well-being of the inmate population is a common goal for both custody and nursing staff, professional frameworks and guiding principles can differ. Nurses in these organizations must be vigilant to maintain professional nursing judgment in all matters of care delivery.

Independent Health Care Service Companies

The next most frequent health care management structure is an independent health care company. Thirty (30) percent of correctional health care is provided through a contracted arrangement between the government entity and a health care company. Nurses are most often employees of the health care service company and report to managers within the company. In this situation, correctional nurses need to understand the contractual relationship with the corrections administration to know what may be required of them. For example, services may include providing health care to security staff and emergency treatment to visitors. Also important is an understanding of the communication and reporting structures among all the players. In this situation, nurses are guests in the facility and must strive to develop collaborative working relationships with custody staff.

A few private companies contract with governments to provide all services in a correctional facility. These companies employ both security and health care staff.

State University Medical Systems

Several state prison systems provide health care to inmates through the state university system. Twelve (12) percent of correctional healthcare is delivered in this manner. For example, in Connecticut inmates receive care through the University of Connecticut medical system and in New Jersey health care services are provided through the state's medical school, Rutger's University. Nurses working in these systems have the advantage of access to academic resources while nursing, medical, and dentistry students have an opportunity to experience the correctional environment. The corollary in jails is that the county health department may provide the health care at the jail. In this situation, nurses have the advantage of access to the resources of the county health department. Although health care staff are not employees of the same entity as corrections staff, a common relationship exists among the government bodies.

Other Correctional Nurse Employers

Nurses may come to practice correctional nursing through other avenues. One area of correctional nursing practice is a locked unit within a community hospital. Hospitals may contract with Departments of Corrections to centralize acute care for inmates. A wing or floor of an acute care facility may be fitted for increased security. All patients on the unit are prisoners from surrounding facilities. Custody officers monitor patients while care is provided by nurses employed by the acute care facility. Similarly, psychiatric facilities may have locked units for the criminally insane.

Nurses may also care for inmate patients as agency or traveling nurses. Many state prisons are located in remote areas far from potential nurse employees. Agency or traveling nurses are engaged for short and long-term assignments at one or several correctional facilities within a system.

The Basics of Caring for Criminals

Providing health care to incarcerated patients is very different than other types of nursing practice; yet nursing principles remain the same. Nurses entering the world of correctional practice can have apprehensions and misconceptions about the patient population and expectations of their practice. Here is an overview of the similarities and differences of correctional nursing practice as compared to a traditional practice setting.

A Different Patient Profile

The inmate patient population has many distinct characteristics to keep in mind when providing care. Although each patient is an individual, the population, as a whole, is likely to have these characteristics that should be taken into consideration when providing care.

- Inmates have a biological age older than their chronological ages. Many experts consider the incarcerated patient to be 10 years older than their chronologic age when it comes to the ravages of age, illness, and lifestyle choices. So, many correctional settings consider elderly inmates to be 50 years and older.

- Less educated and less health literate than the general population, inmates are more likely to have learning disabilities and have difficulty understanding basic health information.

- More infectious diseases, especially HIV, Hepatitis C, sexually transmitted disease, and tuberculosis are found in this patient population.

- Inmates have higher rates of mental illness than the general public, especially depression, mania, and psychotic disorders. Mental illness can contribute to criminality. Borderline personality disorders that lead to poor impulse control, self-injury, and aggression are often present.

- This patient population also has higher rates of traumatic brain injury and post-traumatic stress disorder that can also lead to poor impulse control, erratic behavior, and inability to concentrate or understand health instruction.

- High levels of drug, alcohol, and tobacco use in this population increases the likelihood of withdrawal issues, liver toxicity, and respiratory conditions.

- Increased risk of suicide is found in this patient population as compared to the general population. This is a concern in any stage of the incarceration, but especially of concern at entry into the jail and after sentencing when hopelessness, shame, and guilt are at their highest.

The Same Nursing Care

Nurses enter the correctional facility as licensed in the profession and are expected to provide safe patient care in accordance with that license. This can be challenging in settings where the boundaries of their nursing scope of practice are not clearly defined. Many traditional practice settings are focused only on providing health care and have a strong nursing leadership structure that defines nursing practice within the boundaries of the Nurse Practice Act. Correctional nurses, however, may need to establish their own boundaries of practice; possibly for the first time in their professional career. Three documents provide resources for establishing practice boundaries.

- Nurse Practice Act: Established by the nurse licensing board for the practice jurisdiction (mainly the state of licensure)

- Code of Ethics for Nurses: Established and periodically revised by the American Nurses Association and the International Council of Nurses

- Nursing Scope and Standards of Practice: Established and periodically revised by the American Nurses Association. There are both a general and specialty specific scope and standards of practice.

Nurses are ethically and legally bound to practice within the framework of the profession in every setting. Nurses working in corrections have an acute need to be fully aware of these boundaries as there are fewer safeguards present in our setting.

A Refocused Nursing Perspective

While correctional nurses must practice within the boundaries and responsibilities of licensure, the nursing perspective must be refocused to accommodate a secure setting and a criminal patient population. That means a refocus of care provision to prioritize personal and professional safety.

The first area of refocus is the **nurse-patient relationship**. Although this relationship continues to be based on the health and well-being of the patient, the relationship in the correctional setting must include stronger physical, emotional, and mental boundaries. Caring behaviors cannot include physical touch, as may have been the case in prior nursing positions. Words and actions establish a caring relationship in this setting; not hand-holding, touch, or a shoulder squeeze. The high levels of narcissistic and manipulative personalities within the incarcerated patient population means that nurses must be

27

especially careful to avoid being drawn into an inappropriate patient relationship.

Personal safety is the next area of refocus for correctional nurses. Personal harm from patients is of greater concern when practicing in the criminal justice system. Always be alert when in the work environment. This means being aware of the location of officers and following all facility safety policies and procedures. In a correctional setting, personal safety is of higher priority than immediate emergency care. Thus, correctional nurses must be sure the environment is cleared by officers before entering to provide treatment in an emergency situation such as an unconscious patient in a housing unit.

The final area of practice refocus is **professional safety.** As described earlier, it can be tempting to practice beyond licensure in an isolated and resource-challenged setting such as a jail or prison. It can also be easy to slide into a cynical and jaded attitude to patient requests when so many may be manipulating the system for their own benefit. Yet, overstepping the bounds of licensure or disregarding patient health requests can jeopardize your career and create significant legal risk.

Correctional Nurse Lingo

Every culture and clinical setting has a unique language. Correctional nursing is no exception. Drop into a jail medical unit on a new assignment and you may not be able to follow what is going on. The custody environment and unique medical processes make up the majority of challenges. Many of these terms and abbreviations make their way onto medical charts, causing consternation to the uninitiated. Of course, terms and abbreviations can be regional and/or specific to the facility or state system. Understanding the following terms will jumpstart orientation to a correctional nursing position.

General Abbreviations

BOP: Bureau of Prisons

CO/Officer: Custody Officer: Never refer to officers as guards – very bad form. When known, use rank such as Sargent or Corporal as a sign of respect. Most custody organizations use military rank systems. Other terms used in the criminal justice system include correctional officer or security officer. In jail settings officers may be referred to as deputies.

DOC: Department of Corrections

I/M: Inmate, prisoner, the patient

Inmate Locations

Ad Seg/SHU: Administrative Segregation/Special Housing Unit/Security Housing Unit. Special protective housing or special restrictive housing with less access to or by other inmates. These areas can also isolate inmates from services offered in the general population.

Barracks/Block/Dorm/Pod/Tier: Many names for general population inmate housing areas.

Food Flap/Hatch/Wicket: Knee-level hinged opening in cell door for food delivery and limited access exchanges such as medication administration.

GenPop/Pop/GP: The majority of inmates are in general housing areas without any special protection or accommodations.

SNU: Special Needs Unit. Often a mental health protective unit, this is another restricted area with less access to general facility services, but higher levels of specialized accommodations.

Inmate Items

Contraband: Items prohibited for inmate possession. Contraband lists are specific to facilities and systems. Examples can include cell phones, gum, dental floss, Vaseline, and cigarettes.

Hooch/pruno: Cell-made alcohol from fermented available foods, often fruits.

Shank: Knife created from commonly available materials.

Care Delivery

Chronic Care Clinic: Regularly scheduled appointments to evaluate chronic conditions such as diabetes and hypertension. Mostly physician appointments but may be a nurse appointment for patient education and medication compliance if the condition is stable.

DOT/Watch-Take: Direct-Observation-Therapy.   Medications given in pill line/med line where the inmate is observed taking the medication for compliance and diversion issues.

KOP/On-Person: Keep On Person – medication given to the inmate for self-administration. Reserved for low-risk therapies and medications not deemed of high value on the prison black market.

Kite/Slip/Request: A written request for medical services. Nurses may tell inmates to 'Drop a Slip' or 'Drop a Kite' to obtain an appointment for an evaluation. Requests are triaged based on urgency for the next available appointment.

Med line/Pill line: Medication delivery process. Can take place in the medical unit; in this case, inmates are escorted and lined up in a secure area. Can take place in the housing area; in this case, a nurse rolls the cart to the housing area and inmates line up for medications.

Sick Call: Regularly scheduled access to a nurse or physician. Nurse sick call is usually the first access. A physician appointment is made based on nurse evaluation. Nurses are often able to provide OTC medications based on sick call assessment and pre-approved protocols.

The criminal justice system is based on the military system. Many correctional terms originate from military usage. If you have a military background you will pick up the lingo quickly and be able to navigate and communicate effectively. Even without a military background, you can jumpstart your dialog by using this list of common terms.

Ten Skills You Need as a Correctional Nurse

Correctional nursing practice is unique. According to the Correctional Nursing Scope and Standards of Practice, this specialty is a combination of acute care, emergency, community health, psychiatric, women's health, and palliative care. That is a lot to know about!

On top of that, we often practice in low-resourced settings where we must be a jack-of-all-trades in being able to fulfil a number of roles that are likely delegated to others in a traditional setting. For example, many correctional nurses must be able to draw labs, take an EKG, and give a respiratory treatment.

All of those functions are most often performed by ancillary staff in an acute care setting. Nurses entering the correctional specialty may need to brush up on or develop new skill in the following areas.

Dental Assessment

Who knew we would need to deal with teeth as nurses? Yet many a nursing sick call request is tooth-related. Become friends with the site dentist and ask for help and mentoring in dental assessment skills. Of particular importance is the ability to differentiate when a dental request needs immediate referral to the dentist and when it can await the next available dental appointment.

Ear Assessment

There are plenty of ear infections to evaluate among the correctional patient population. This requires the ability to handle an otoscope and understand what is observed. Seek out a nurse practitioner or other experienced staff for mentoring.

Electrocardiogram (EKG)

Is that sudden onset chest pain described by an otherwise healthy 38 year-old patient a cardiac, gastrointestinal, or behavioral condition? A 12-lead EKG will help with diagnosis if the leads are placed correctly. How about reading the output? Is there instant access to outside EKG reading services or must a copy of the EKG be faxed to the on-call provider? In any case, fundamental understanding of 12-lead EKG operation and interpretation are needed in most correctional settings.

Labor, Delivery, and Fetal Heart Tones

Pregnant women in jails and prisons are likely to be at high risk for premature deliveries or complications. Many times correctional nurses must evaluate symptoms of labor onset and fetal health. Occasionally, a precipitous delivery requires in-cell management.

Phlebotomy

Starting an IV is one thing, drawing tubes of blood is something else. Add to that, drawing labs on an IV drug user and things get difficult really fast. And that doesn't even take into account determining which tubes to use, which need to spin down, and which need refrigeration until pick up.

Physical Therapy

In many correctional settings nurses act as adjuncts to Physical Therapists in managing the patient on the prescribed physical therapy regimen. Nurses may need to reinforce PT teaching, monitor exercises, and chart patient progress in mobility and function.

Respiratory Treatments and Oxygen Tanks

Although basic nebulizer treatments are not difficult to administer, many nurses do not have experience administering them as they are often administered by respiratory therapists in traditional settings. Reviewing basic technique may be necessary.

Likewise, wall oxygen is rare and oxygen tanks are the norm in most correctional settings. Heavy metal pressurized oxygen tanks can be a safety issue. Orientation as to how to 'crack' the tank and initiate oxygen flow may be needed.

Skin Issues: Inflammation, Infections, Infestations

Correctional nurses are called upon to evaluate many skin conditions and need to be able to effectively describe what is seen as well as determine if the condition needs Provider attention. Whether determining MRSA, scabies, or a suspicious mole, skin issues are big in the correctional specialty! Start now developing skill in identifying what you see as well as documenting it. Infestations with lice, bed bugs, or scabies are also common in the incarcerated patient population, so early identification and treatment is important to community health.

Splints, Slings, Casts

Having an emergency nursing background can be very helpful when dealing with orthopedic patient injuries common in correctional facilities. Splints, slings, and even casting may be part of correctional nursing activities. A basic first aid course can be a valuable addition to your training. A link to a 3M playlist of basic casting and splinting can be found at correctionalnurse.net/quickstart.

TB Skin Testing: Placement and Reading

Proper placement and correct reading of Mantoux tuberculin skin tests (TST) is a specialized skill given only brief treatment in most nursing school programs and infrequently used by most nurses in traditional health care roles. Yet, correctional nurses are often required to place and read a TST on every incoming inmate.

Visual Acuity Testing

Right up there with teeth, ears, and skin is the need to evaluate vision and eye conditions in correctional nursing practice. Visual acuity evaluation may be needed after eye trauma or at intake screening. The standard Snellen eye chart is most frequently used in correctional assessments. Nurses need to understand the correct process for administering and documenting a visual acuity exam.

There are many more nursing skills needed by correctional nurses but this is a priority list of less-familiar skills that can jumpstart a correctional nurse skill development program.

How to Work with Correctional Officers

In most settings where nurses practice, the interdisciplinary team includes other health care professionals such as physicians, diagnostic technicians, and pharmacists. Sure, there may be unlicensed ancillary staff in the mix such as admissions clerks and supply personnel, but everyone is generally focused on the goal of providing health care. Not so in a correctional facility. Here, in addition to other health care professionals, correctional nurses also collaborate and negotiate with correctional officers as legitimate members of the health care team. It is a mistake to minimize the impact of good communication among nurses and officers on safe patient outcomes. Armed with an understanding of the correctional officer role and responsibilities, correctional nurses can successfully advance inmate health care in a correctional setting.

Officers are Professionals, Too

If you are a team sport enthusiast, you know that everyone on the sports team has a position to play and each player needs to play their position, as well as understand the role of other team players. It is no different for the correctional health care team. Everyone has a role to play and it is important to both understand and acknowledge the different perspectives between security and health care. Correctional officers are professionals in their field and their perspective is important to many of the health care decisions needed for the patient population.

There are likely to be philosophical differences between the two disciplines, though, and it is important for correctional nurses to develop a keen understanding of the security perspective in order to successfully advocate for a patient's health needs. Most of these differences come from different orientations; officers are taught that security and rule compliance is paramount, while nurses are taught that caring and compassion is paramount. The truth is - both are right. Some call this the custody-caring friction between the security and nursing perspectives. It may be a difficult adjustment to learn to work with officers without sacrificing a nursing perspective on the patient population. For example, officers may be critical of nursing concepts like compassion and patient advocacy. Their ethical framework is less bound by the nursing concepts of caring, advocacy, and human dignity. However, honesty, justice, and civil rights are all part of most professional codes, so there is strong overlap between the professions.

Correctional officers are professionals, too, and deserve respectful treatment. Nurses who are arrogant or act superior to their correctional colleagues don't last in the specialty. We may come from different worldviews and we may have differing opinions, but both professions have a vital role in the facility. The happiest correctional nurses are those who build collegial relationships with the officers with whom they work.

Aretha was Right – R-E-S-P-E-C-T

Civil and respectful communication and behavior among the disciplines is the secret to collaborative success. This means respecting the role officers play in successful health care outcomes. Nurses can role model respectfulness even if custody officers are less than civil in return. This, of course, is difficult, but can also be empowering and powerful. In a culture of disrespect, respectful behavior stands out.

It is important to acknowledge and respect the security perspective without internalizing or modeling it. Correctional nurses are not custody officers and should not try to be so. As stated earlier, each team member has a role to play and should not try to play the position of other team members. Unfortunately, some nurses slide into a custody mindset without realizing it. It is helpful to regularly and mindfully re-center your thoughts to your role as healer. It may be helpful to establish a ritual where this mindfulness takes place as you daily enter the security checkpoint.

Security personnel are like most people – they have preconceived notions about how nurses behave and think. Sometimes, correctional staff can be critical of nursing concepts like compassion and patient advocacy, but they still do not like it when nurses do not act as expected. Role modeling expected nurse behavior may invite some teasing, but generally the security staff will have greater respect for the nurses who remain true to their professional values.

When Asked to Do Something that is Out-of-Bounds

Officers don't always know what nurses do and may have misconceptions about what can be asked of a nurse. If unprepared for these requests or unknowledgeable about licensure boundaries, correctional nurses can end up practicing outside practice boundaries in an attempt to be helpful.

Have a well-thought-out response for when you are asked by an officer or security administrator to perform a function that is outside your professional or ethical boundaries. Remember, these folks may not know they are asking you to do something unlawful or unethical. Give them the benefit of the doubt. Here is an example to get you started thinking about how you can respond respectfully and collegially. "I'd really like to help you out with this issue but what you are asking me to do is beyond what my nursing license allows (or is not considered ethical for a nurse to do). Let's see if we can come up with a solution that works for all of us." Having a prepared response will ease the stress of declining a request and start the discussion toward a solution.

HIPAA and Officer Need-to-Know

Although it is important to consider correctional officers as part of the health care team, their legal access to patient health information is limited. Officers, however, do require information about an inmate's health status when it is needed for the inmate's health or for the health and safety of staff and the inmate population. Many times you need to enlist the help of a correctional officer. They can be your eyes and ears in the housing unit; if you ask them.

That means officers may need to know about medical conditions or disabilities that require special equipment or scheduled appointments. Some medication side effects require additional attention or changes in the inmate's work duty. Joint surgery may limit movements or abilities that security needs to be aware of. Fortunately, the Health Insurance Portability and Accountability Act (HIPAA) regulations take into account the need for some information sharing within the correctional setting and have spelled this out in the 45 C.F.R. 164.512 (k) (5) (i) section of the code. A link to the full document can be found at correctinalnurse.net/quickstart.

HIPAA permits disclosure to correctional institutions if this protected health information is necessary for any of the following.

• The provision of health care to such individuals

• The health and safety of such individuals or other inmates

• The health and safety of the officers or employees, or of others at the correctional institution

• The health and safety of such individuals and officers or other persons responsible for the transporting of inmates or their transfer from one institution, facility, or setting to another

- Law enforcement on the premises of the correctional institution

- The administration and maintenance of the safety, security, and good order of the correctional institution

Generally speaking, avoid discussing specifics about a patient's medical or mental health conditions with officers except in these situations.

- Officers need to be alert to an urgent need of medical attention such as an unstable diabetic, seizure disorder, or post-concussion mental status

- The condition needs special housing or activity interventions such as pregnancy, back injury, or joint replacement

- The patient is allergic to a common element in the environment or diet such as peanut butter or bee sting

If in doubt about the need or the advisability of communicating particular health information, seek guidance from the health supervisor or medical director. Be sure the information shared can be supported by one of the six necessity requirements listed above.

With a focus on maintaining professional nursing integrity while also understanding the correctional officer perspective, most nurses can successfully negotiate the caring-custody divide and establish a collegial and respectful relationship with officers at their facility.

Potential Interview Questions

Preparing for an interview for a correctional nursing position includes developing honest and thoughtful answers to potential interview questions. If this is your first correctional experience, it may be difficult to know what questions are commonly asked and also difficult to spontaneously respond to unfamiliar areas of questioning. Listed here and grouped by general themes are common questions that may be asked on a phone or in-person correctional nurse job interview.

Questions about Working in Corrections

The interviewer is likely to ask about why you are applying to work in a correctional setting. Think through your motivation for the position and develop an honest and positive response to questions like these.

Why do you want to work in a correctional facility?

Develop some positive and constructive answers to this question. Some possibilities might be enjoying a challenge, desiring to work in a close-knit team, enjoying variety in the type of care delivered and making an impact on a needy and disadvantaged population. As correctional health care is based on public health principles, an interest in public health can also be included in your answer. Choose one or two reasons and develop a 3-4 sentence response.

How do you feel about providing care for inmates?

This is a good question to ponder before you apply for a position in corrections. The environment is challenging and you want to be sure there is a good match. Many who thrive in the corrections specialty consider their role in caring for the disadvantaged or their impact on public health.

It is perfectly acceptable to share that you are a bit nervous about working behind bars. Your interviewer will expect a bit of anxiety but, if you are immobilized by fear and apprehension, this setting is not for you.

Describe your background in nursing and how this will complement the duties for a correctional nurse.

Working in corrections involves medication administration, patient teaching, ambulatory care visits, emergency response, therapeutic communication and dealing with behavior and psychiatric issues. Think carefully through your past nursing experiences and have a story or two to share about your background that highlights one or more of these areas.

Questions about Working with Inmates

Manipulative behavior is very common among the inmate population. What are some nursing skills that are helpful in dealing with this behavior?

Correctional nurses must be able to deliver necessary nursing care and remain objective in evaluating symptoms and patient concerns. Ponder any prior patient situations where you handled manipulation to provide an example. Key nursing actions to minimize manipulation are to set clear and firm limits and to let the patient know that that you know and follow security rules.

What would you do if an inmate asked you for a favor? What if an inmate gives you a letter to mail on the outside?

Incarcerated patients may attempt to use the nurse-patient relationship to circumvent facility rules. Like the response for manipulative behavior, the nurse needs to be firm, fair, and consistent. The response to a request for a favor such as mailing a letter (which is completely against security policy) is to identify that the request is inappropriate and guide the conversation back to the health issue at hand. A single request may be boundary checking on the part of the inmate. Continual requests for favors should be reported to your supervisor.

While potential employees will not be expected to know all facility rules during the interview, awareness that even the most banal inmate request might not be allowed in prison needs to be acknowledged.

How do you maintain boundaries with manipulative patients?

Do some reading about manipulative behavior and professional nursing boundaries. Develop ideas for responding to this behavior from inmates – it is pervasive. Generally, combat manipulative behavior by being alert to it and responding in a firm, fair, and consistent manner. Also, treat all inmate-patients with professional respect. Discuss the importance of staying within the zone of helpfulness in the nurse-patient relationship and avoiding straying into a personal relationship. Acknowledge that correctional nurses must be ever mindful of professional practice boundaries.

What would you do if, while administering medications, the patient throws the pills and water back at you?

Dealing with inmate behavior issues is a part of life in many correctional settings, so some form of question like this may be asked during an interview. Again, search back in your past experiences for a similar episode with a patient. If you remember one, share it and your response. Otherwise, key concepts to have in your response are to:

- Remain calm

- Consider the context of this action (is the patient already known to be agitated, mentally ill, or aggressive?)

- Try to determine the cause of the outburst by engaging the patient in a conversation, if appropriate

- Document and communicate the medication refusal

- Check on the critical nature of the medication

- Report incident as required by institutional policy

Questions about Your Nursing Experiences

Questions about your nursing experiences are a part of any position interview, no matter the specialty. They are included here to help you prepare for a well-rounded interview. Focus on the relationship of your experience as they might relate to the unique setting and patient population of correctional health care.

You have 60 seconds - tell me about yourself.

The interviewer is looking for a self-appraisal as a nurse, so limit your hobbies and interests here unless they might give insight to your values or motivation. For example, if you volunteer at a homeless shelter, that might be of interest. Otherwise, prepare a short response to a question like this that focuses on honest positives about yourself that fit the role of a correctional nurse (based on information from this book).

Describe a specific time you knew you were in over your head with a patient, what you did about it, and what you learned from the experience.

You are likely to be in over your head at some point in your correctional practice. The interviewer wants to hear that you remained level-headed and made wise decisions about how to solve the situation. Think back on your nursing career for a specific example and emphasize how you initiated action, sought out assistance, and kept the patient safe. Be sure to include what you learned from the experience. It can be a confirmation of something you did in the experience. It does not need to be an acknowledgement that you didn't do something you should have.

47

Describe a specific time you had difficulty with a patient's behavior, how you handled it, and what you learned from the situation.

Correctional health care is full of patients with anger management issues and poor behavior control. The interviewer wants to know that you can deal with difficult patient behavior. Like the prior question, prepare a response that describes an actual patient experience you had and how you managed it. It doesn't need to be a complicated situation. Something as simple as a patient being upset that his pain medication was delayed will work.

Name a specific example of a time you were reprimanded at work, how you handled it and what you learned.

Here the interviewer wants to know that you are willing to take corrective feedback and use it to improve your nursing practice. If you have never been reprimanded at work, state this and, instead, share a story of when you received a constructive critique during a performance review or critical incident. Emphasize your desire to excel in nursing practice and that you thoughtfully consider all feedback in order to make improvements in future practice.

Give a specific example of a time you had multiple things to do, all at the same time. How did you prioritize your tasks and what did you learn?

This is a common example question for all nursing positions. Correctional nursing requires prioritizing and re-prioritizing activities throughout the shift. Develop a good example of how you did that in a difficult situation. Things to include might be pausing to re-evaluate the situation, considering the most important actions to take immediately based on patient acuity and safety, and seeking out opportunities for delegation.

If you were up against someone with the same level of education and experience for this position, tell me why I should hire you over someone else.

When compared equally to another applicant on education and experience, your advantage can lie in your motivation, values, and even flexibility. For example, you may have a desire to work with a disadvantaged or behaviorally challenging patient population. Although you may have the same years of experience as another applicant, your experience might be better suited to the correctional setting and patient population. You may be able to say that you are a flexible worker and willing to work a variety of shifts or positions. Develop a list of ways you are more than your education and experience so you can answer a question like this one.

What would your current supervisor say if we asked what your strengths and weaknesses were?

This can be a challenging question to answer; especially if you and your current supervisor do not see things in the same way. That is why it is good to be prepared for this question and answer it confidently. There are multiple perspectives on a situation and you want to present the most positive perspective on your strengths and weaknesses. Do you have philosophical differences with your supervisor? That can mean that you are guided by your values, determined, and forthright.

Have you been reprimanded by your supervisor? If so, consider how you responded to the critique. Can you say that you take constructive criticism well? Be sure to have a response that includes both strengths and weaknesses as the interviewer is likely to probe further if you do not offer both.

Describe a situation when you were forced to make a decision that no one else agreed with.

Correctional nurses can sometimes be in a situation where there is a need to make a decision that no one else agrees with. It could be an urgent need for the patient to be transported to the hospital or it could be the need to address an emerging ethical issue. The interviewer wants to know that you will be able to overcome obstacles in order to get the care needed for the patient, even if no one else agrees with you. Ponder situations in your past experience where you needed to persuade others of the right course of action and develop a list of actions you took to accomplish your objective.

Questions about Nursing Care

Nursing in a correctional facility requires specialized skills, knowledge and work behaviors. Describe what you think they are.

Skills might include excellent objective assessment, communication, emergency response, and organization skills to shift gears quickly while still getting required work done. Knowledge might include understanding of communicable diseases, the health needs of the inmate population, and safety procedures. Work behaviors would include being reliable, always letting team members know where you are, good follow-through, and being firm, fair and consistent with inmates and staff.

How would you do patient teaching for an inmate on how to manage diabetes?

In answering any question about patient teaching, be sure to mention the need to present the material in easy-to-understand language. In addition, be sure to note that some patients may not be able to read, making written material less helpful. It is good to include the teach-back method where patients are asked to repeat back what they have learned to determine retention (Kripalani, Bengtzen, Henderson, & Jacobson, 2008).

Name some psychotropic drugs and their side effects.

Incarcerated patients have high levels of mental illness including depression, psychosis, and personality disorders. That means plenty of psychotropic drug administration and side effect management. Brush up on common psyche meds and their side effects for a possible interview question like this one.

What would you do if you found an unresponsive or unconscious inmate?

The important concern in corrections is always safety. Therefore, your response would be to summon help and proceed only after custody officers indicate that it is safe to begin care. It seems counter-intuitive to wait, but with the inmate population you need to be sure you are secure before assisting someone. Of course, once safety has been established you would initiate all the standard emergency medical assessments and procedures like airway, breathing, circulation, etc.

How do you think your nursing practice will change when you come to work in this jail/prison?

Here the interviewer wants assurance that you plan to practice according to professional standards in a correctional setting just as you would in a traditional health setting. Confirm that you would practice according to the Nurse Practice Act, Scope and Standards of Practice, and the Code of Ethics for Nurses. Then identify that the unique environment and patient population provides a different context for nursing care and this context would create the health conditions and processes of care. These would be different and would constitute the changes in your practice.

General Nursing Questions

Interviewers often want to confirm general nursing knowledge for common correctional nursing processes. Be prepared to answer questions about your standard systems for the following common nursing activities.

- Medication administration – 5 Rights
- Hand hygiene and infection control
- Nursing assessment
- Emergency response

Disease-Related Questions

The interviewer may ask questions related to common conditions and diseases prevalent in the correctional patient population. Perform an internet search or pull out a basic nursing text and brush up on these conditions.

- Abdominal pain
- Chest pain
- Heat exhaustion/Heat stroke
- Hepatitis
- HIV
- Hyper and hypoglycemia
- Narcotics overdose
- Orthopedic issues - sprains, strains, fractures
- Respiratory distress
- Skin conditions – athlete's Foot/eczema
- Tuberculosis

What to Know Before You Go to the Interview

As you prepare for an on-site interview at a correctional facility, you will want to know how to negotiate entry into a secure setting. Correctional facilities are arranged to keep the inmates inside and to keep out unwanted individuals and material that can be used inappropriately if obtained by inmates. Here are some things to ask, consider, and plan for when preparing for on on-site interview at a correctional facility.

What to Ask

Don't be afraid to ask what to expect. Although there are similarities across the various types of facilities and levels of security, there is also great variability as to focus.

Each security culture has its own peculiarities. Even within a state prison system, some facilities may be stricter than others. You will want to be prepared. Ask if someone will meet you at the door (recommended). Find out their name, position, and telephone extension. If they are not there when you arrive, give this information to the reception officer so an escort arrangement can be made.

Ask about what to wear and what you can bring into the facility. Below are some general rules for consideration.

What to Wear

Clothing serves many purposes in corrections. Clothing designates the status of many of the officers and staff in the custody profession. Clothing also designates the inmate population in many facilities. Inmates must often relinquish personal possessions during intake and are provided standard issue jumpsuits or 'uniforms'. The standard color for inmate wear is usually off-limits for staff apparel. Find out what those colors are and be sure not to be wearing them or you may be prohibited entry. Correctional facilities also often require modest dress. For example, some facilities do not allow sleeveless tops and most do not allow low or even moderately low necklines. The determination may be at the discretion of the entry staff. Don't take chances before you know the culture. Dress conservatively for an interview.

Many places do not allow open-toe shoes or jewelry. Hoop earrings and necklaces can be used to harm and even kill the wearer. Another clothing challenge for females is the underwire bra. The wire stays provide excellent support but often activate the security alarm at the staff entrance. You may need to switch out your undies collection for your new position.

What to Bring

Like clothing, approved personal items that can be brought into a facility can also vary. For example, some facilities do not allow any food brought in, others do not allow liquids or anything made of glass. Still others allow liquids if unopened and in plastic bottles. Cell phones and other electronics are almost universally banned. Some facilities require all carry bags to be of clear plastic so that all items are visible for inspection. Keep it simple and pare down your required personal carry items. Bring your driver's license, keys, and any paperwork with you.

What to Expect at the Door

You will most definitely have a security check at the entrance to the facility. This usually includes passing through a metal detector and possibly a pat-down. The pat-down should be done by a same-gender officer. Personal items not allowed in the facility are best left in your locked car, but many facilities also have lockers at the entrance for small items. There will also be a log book to sign and date when entering and leaving the facility. This information is useful if there is a need to evacuate the facility or account for all individuals in a potential hostage situation.

With thoughtful planning, you will breeze through your first security check. In no time, these principles will be an automatic part of your correctional nursing practices.

Preparing for the Interview: Calming Interview Anxiety

You've landed a correctional nurse job interview and spent the last few days preparing responses to common correctional nurse interview questions. You drove to the site at about the same time of day as the upcoming interview, located where to park, and set up tomorrow's schedule to get to the interview 30 minutes early to account for the entry process. You even called ahead to get information about dress code and security procedure for entering the facility. You have prepared as best as you can, but now your anxiety is spiraling out of control as you try to sleep the evening before that big day. How will you ever get a good night's rest so that your mind will be clear to answer those questions?

Job interviews are anxiety producing; especially if you really need or want that position. Here are some tips from the experts on how to calm anxieties and do your best at your correctional nurse interview.

General Preparation

- Recognize that interview anxiety is normal and most people are keyed up before an important performance.

- Understand that an interview is like a stage performance; except that you are not playing a part but are presenting your very best 'you' in the situation.

- Take deep breaths and meditate on calming scenes, past successful situations, helpful quotations, or Bible verses.

- Do not focus on past failures or mistakes. They are history and don't define who you are. Let them go.

- Instead, focus on the future, and imagine yourself leaving the facility being delighted with the interview discussion.

- Don't schedule an important activity directly after the interview so you don't add anxiety about missing or needing to re-schedule that event.

Day of the Interview

- Eat a light breakfast, even if you aren't hungry. Food helps your brain function.

- Rehydrate with fluid in the morning but don't overdo the caffeine. A little is good. A lot will put you on edge.

- Wear comfortable yet professional clothing. Include comfortable walking shoes as you may have a distance to go to get to the medical unit once inside the security perimeter.

- Bring your cell phone and have the number of the interviewer handy. If something unexpected delays you, contacting the interviewer will be paramount.

During the Interview

- Focusing on hiding your anxiety will only help escalate it. Instead, focus on truly listening to the interviewer's questions and developing an appropriate answer.

- Instead of thinking of the meeting as an interview or interrogation, consider it a conversation where you and the interviewer are focused on the goal of meeting a need.

- In between answers, breathe deeply. This can slow your heart rate and quiet your mind. You can practice this on your trip to the facility.

- Don't speed into answering a question, even if it is one you prepared for and have a great answer for. Pause to organize your thoughts and then speak. If you are prone to rapid speech when anxious, work on slowing down your sentences.

- Pay attention to your posture. Sitting upright gives a confident presentation.

- Bring an extra resume, note paper, and a pencil. Have your schedule in mind in case a follow-up interview is arranged. You will likely not be able to enter with a cell phone so an electronic calendar will not be available to you.

Calming anxiety can go a long way toward being your best in a job interview. Include managing your anxiety as part of your interview prep activities.

How to Spot a Good Place to Work

So you are thinking about correctional nursing and even have an interview set up at a local facility. Besides preparing yourself to be at your best for the interview, consider how you will determine if this correctional setting is a good place for you to work. There are three important components of a quality correctional health care setting.

- Personal Safety

- Professional Safety

- Collegiality and Collaboration

Even though you prepare for your interview with the idea of a job offer in mind, you also want to fully evaluate whether you will be safe and able to work effectively in the setting. You also want to determine your emotional response to being behind bars. Some nurses are unnerved by the security process or the number of locked doors they must pass through before reaching the medical unit. Be mindful of your surroundings and your emotional response as you are escorted to the interview location.

Personal Safety

During your security entry, take note of the diligence with which the officers perform their duties. You want to know that they follow procedure and are not lax in their position. If their focus is on chatting or other non-work activities, they may be distracted from their primary role - your safety.

Be sure to get a full tour of the facility, including every location in which you may be working as a staff nurse. Pay attention to the number and location of custody staff at each location. There should be an officer available at all times for security purposes. When touring the care delivery areas, take note of the layout of the area and how staff access officers when at risk. For example, are there alarm buttons in rooms or are staff always within hearing distance of security staff? Note how many security staff are available and if they have multiple duties or distractions. They should be attentive to what is going on in the unit.

During the interview you will be asked for any questions you might have. Take this opportunity to find out the following:

- *Does nurse orientation include orientation to security procedures and dealing with inmates?* A good orientation in corrections includes more than policy and procedure. You will want to hear that you would receive information about security procedures, how to remain safe in the facility, safety codes and rules, as well as how to deal with the inmate population.

- *Are nurses given safety alarm mechanisms? What is used in this facility?* There should be a mechanism for nurses to sound an alarm if they feel they are in an unsafe situation. Generally, staff will not be out of sight and/or sound of a custody officer at any time. However, even with mirrors for 'blind spots' there is a small opportunity for loss of contact. A well-run facility will have a mechanism in place to alert security to an unsafe situation.

- *What is the procedure for nurse movement in the inmate areas of the facility?* The safest procedure is an officer escort, but some settings may allow staff members to travel from checkpoint to checkpoint. Staff should not travel alone in areas where there may be direct contact with inmates.

Professional Safety

Being safe from physical harm is a priority for working in a correctional setting, but professional jeopardy is also important. Professional safety involves the level of risk to your license and professional integrity. Professional practice is bound by the Nurse Practice Act, the Scope and Standards of Practice, and the Code of Ethics for Nurses (full links at corrrectionalnurse.net/quickstart). Since correctional facilities are not primarily health care sites, some settings may not have sufficient nursing structure to support safe professional practice. It may be difficult to observe professional safety in place during a facility tour, but questions can be asked that will help determine professional risk.

- *Who will I report to in this position?* If the medical unit manager is not a nurse, there should be a registered nurse with responsibility for nursing practice issues. This might be a Director of Nursing at the facility or a Regional Director of Nursing with oversight for several facilities.

- *What is the procedure if I have a nursing practice issue?* Nursing practice issues need to be resolved through nursing leadership. Unlicensed managers or correctional leaders are not equipped to make nursing practice decisions.

- *What levels of staff will I be working with and delegating to?* This question will help you determine if delegation to LP/VNs or unlicensed assistive personnel is required.

- *What is the procedure if I see unethical health care practice or unethical treatment of patients by correctional staff?* Many correctional nurses find themselves witnessing unethical practices among officers and health care staff. It is important to know that there is a process for reporting and ending unethical practices.

- *Is the facility accredited by the National Commission on Correctional Health Care (NCCHC) or the American Correctional Associations (ACA)?* Current accreditation with either of these independent bodies indicates that the facility meets nationally recognized quality standards. Their seal of approval is similar to a Joint Commission accreditation for hospitals. An accredited facility is more likely to have well running clinical processes and established practices.

Collegiality and Collaboration

Good correctional health care is nearly impossible without the cooperation of officers and correctional leadership. While taking the facility tour, observe how nurses and officers interact in the housing areas and medical unit. Is the atmosphere tense or friendly? Are nursing requests met with equanimity or disdain? What does the body language tell you about the nature of the relationship among the disciplines in the organization? Additional questions can also be asked about communication among the disciplines.

- *Do the officers consider nurses to be colleagues or guests in the facility?* In a smooth-working facility, health care staff are considered part of operations rather than a guest. Guest status may seem preferable. After all, in a hospitality situation, guests are often treated better and with more courtesy than family. However, guest status in a correctional facility can mean health care staff are unable to negotiate for or advocate for patient health care. In a secure setting, guests who don't comply with the status quo can be escorted out of the facility and banned from return.

- *If I had an issue with an officer about a patient's health need that couldn't be resolved, what would be the next step?* Correctional nurses must respectfully collaborate with officer peers regarding the health needs of the patient population. When an important

66

patient health issue cannot be resolved at the peer level, there needs to be a mechanism to engage various levels of leadership until a mutually satisfying solution is found.

Interviewing for a nursing position at an unfamiliar correctional setting is as much about evaluating the work environment as it is about being evaluated for a good fit for the position. Take time during the interview process to determine the level of personal safety, professional safety, and collegiality in the organization. Armed with this information you can decide how you want to answer when you get that job offer!

Job, Career, or Calling
– It's Up to You!

"It's not what you look at that matters, it's what you see"
– Henry David Thoreau

So, is correctional nursing for you? It can be! If you are looking for a challenging and fulfilling opportunity to provide nursing care, you may need to look no further than your closest jail or prison. Most of us enter nursing to help others in need. There is no needier patient population than those in the criminal justice system.

Correctional nursing can be a job, a career, or a calling based on your perspective – what do you see?

- If you see your work life as an endless string of shiftwork, passing pills and triaging sick call slips, then you may have a **job** perspective

- If you see your work life as a stepping stone to an advanced position, then you may have a **career** focus

- If you see your work life as meaningful to the lives of others and personally fulfilling, then you may have a **calling** focus

Those who research job satisfaction found that those who see their work as a calling do work they care about. They consider their work to be more than a means to an end, but an opportunity to find meaning and do something important. These researchers also found that those who viewed their work as a calling were healthier, had greater satisfaction with their life and missed less work than those in either the Job or Career categories.

Knowing your work orientation can help you find ways to motivate yourself and craft a better work situation without having to change jobs. Job crafting, in fact, is a primary way correctional nurses can move from a Job perspective to a Calling perspective regarding their work life.

Dimensions of Meaning

Experts have determined five dimensions of meaning that can be found in work.

- **Money:** Although correctional nursing salaries can be competitive, it is not one of the highest paying nursing specialties.

- **Status:** Correctional nursing practice has made advances of the last decade, but nurses working in jails and prisons can still be stigmatized by their patient population and work setting.

- **Making a difference:** Correctional nurses can make a significant contribution to the health and well-being of a marginalized and disadvantaged patient group.

- **Following your passions:** What motivated you to become a nurse? How would that align with correctional nursing practice?

- **Using your talents:** Many passions also end up being talents. What nursing talents do you have that are applied in a correctional nursing position?

What is Job Crafting?

Job crafting is a way to redesign work perspective, relationships, and tasks to improve job satisfaction. Job boundaries can expand or contract over time based on the individual in the position and the aspects that are emphasized or de-emphasized. It starts with determining the areas of a role that are the most meaningful, provide the most satisfaction, and are aligned with gifts and talents. While in many situations other areas of the role cannot be neglected, focusing on extending time and effort toward gaining experience and expertise in areas of fulfillment craft the position.

Ways to Job Craft

Even in the most structured of job descriptions, there is room for modifications to make work life more satisfying and meaningful. Researchers found that successful job crafters took action in three areas: perspective, relationships, and tasks. Here are some suggestions specific to a correctional nursing role.

- **Perspective:** It all starts in the mind. Mentally seeing your work as affecting the lives and health of your patients is more helpful than seeing your work as a list of nursing tasks that must be completed by the end of the shift. Thus, correctional nursing is not medication administration, sick call, emergency response, and intake screening but "the protection of health, prevention of illness and injury, and alleviation of suffering" (definition from the Correctional Nursing Scope and Standards of Practice, 2013). Successful job crafters reframe the social purpose of their positions to align with their values and concerns. What parts of the definition of correctional nursing do you highly value? Be mindful of those themes during your day-to-day activities.

- **Relationships:** The type and extent of relationship with various workmates can be a way to craft a more positive work experience. Hang around unhappy, stressed, and cynical people and you will find yourself mirroring their moods and emotions (Lewandowski, 2012). The reverse is also true. Honestly evaluate the perspective of each member of your work team and develop deeper relationship with those who will encourage and facilitate your highly valued role components.

- **Tasks:** Evaluate which elements of the correctional nursing role give you the most pleasure and fulfillment. Ponder the specific themes of these elements. For example, if you enjoy sick call, which parts? Is it the assessment, the patient interaction, the teaching component? Find ways to do more of the satisfying component. That might not mean the original job task. For example, if assessment is the satisfying part of the sick call process then intake screening is also a task that would provide opportunity for more assessment. If patient teaching is the driving satisfier then chronic care tasks may be an additional option. Once determined, seek ways to increase satisfying tasks while decreasing or streamlining less valued tasks to accommodate the change.

Just a Job? Just a Step in the Ladder? Just a Way to Make a Difference?

So, what will it be for you? Will correctional nursing be just a job that meets your monthly bills and is available until you find something better? Is the position just a step on the career path to a position of more power and prestige? Or, is correctional nursing a way that you can make a difference in the lives of others, creating a meaningful professional life of compassion and service? In the end, it is up to you.

"We don't see things the way they are, we see things the way we are." – Anais Nin

APPENDIX

Tales from Jails (and Prisons) Around the Country

When considering a position in a new specialty, it can be helpful to hear stories from nurses who have worked in the specialty. This is an opportunity to get a better understanding both of how nurses practice in the criminal justice system and how they make a difference for their patient population.

My Story

Mary Loos, BSN, MPH, spent her correctional nursing career in the Multnomah County Health Department, providing care in the Multnomah County Jail System.

Every person who discovers Corrections Health as a career has their own story to tell about how they got there. Mine? It started with a right turn in my path to work in the Public Health arena. After earning my BSN, I decided to get RN experience for a year or two. Before I knew it, I had spent 14 years in hospital nursing, working my way up from staff nurse to hospital nursing supervisor. My clinical experience provided me with a wealth of experience in pediatrics, general and vascular surgery, post-op open heart / telemetry, quick decision-making and working with many different disciplines.

In 1985, I realized that I didn't want to work in a hospital anymore. The first time I looked in the local newspaper for a nursing position, I saw an ad for a Nurse Manager position in our county's Corrections Health program within the Public Health Department. My mind started making the connection right away – the public's health includes all sectors of the population. I immediately completed an application for this position, toured facilities and had several interviews. I was hired to work with a person I soon realized was a visionary and a national leader in the Corrections Health professional arena.

At last, I was in Public Health! And that is the way my Program Director and I, along with our entire team, carried our mission out. We grew from three facilities to six, doubling our census of patients between the years I was there. We dealt with the onset of AIDS and the corresponding issues of confidentiality and safety precautions, which was an extremely sensitive issue with custody and program staff. Our infirmaries grew along with higher complexity patients, our

74

funding cycles went up and down, and threats of litigation motivated all staff to chart precisely and timely. Interdisciplinary challenges aside, I found working in this environment stimulating, educational, and truly worthwhile.

We established many joint public health programs within the jail facilities. Among these was our participation in a joint project with community corrections and community health, ensuring that drug-addicted pregnant women in custody were connected with community health nurses both in and out of custody. We also set up an official Food Handler Certificate program for inmates, putting them one step closer to a job on release. Corrections Health has evolved over the years into a high technology program that provides basic and complex care to a population that rotates in and out rapidly, and often arrive in booking with unstable and/or acute symptoms. The staff is incredible – experienced, knowledgeable, skilled, compassionate yet limit-setting, and they juggle a patient load that no other health care personnel face.

And yes, I've had people ask why I'm not working as a "real nurse", and why am I working with "those people". My response was unswerving: that I've chosen to work with a microcosm of our county population that is sicker due to lack of consistent medical and mental health care. They, like us, need and deserve health care. This has led to some interesting conversations, I assure you. Corrections Health is Public Health at its best. Once you enter the field, it's easy to get hooked, and longevity in this elite field is common. You either hate it and leave, or you love it and stay. To this day, the years I worked with jail inmates are the highlight of my 42-year nursing career.

Something's Not Right Here

Laura Mish, RN, works in a medium security prison with an average daily population of 3,300 male inmates. Here is one of her correctional nursing tales.

The Background

Having been a correctional nurse at a state prison for nearly 16 years, I have many stories to tell. Some are sad, some are funny, and then there are those that you will never forget. They change your perspective, not only on correctional nursing, but on nursing in general. I have learned invaluable lessons from many of my inmate patients, and I would like to share one with you.

The Tale

Several years ago, while working one of the medical units in general population, I received a call from one of the officers on a housing unit. It was just past 2pm, which is change of shift for medical as well as security staff. The officer told me that he had an inmate that was complaining of a headache. He said the headache was his only complaint, but that it was getting worse as the day went on. Thinking that this was going to be a fairly easy emergency sick call, I told the officer to send him down.

While I was waiting for him to arrive, I reviewed his medical record and noted that he was rarely in medical for any issues, and had no current medical diagnoses listed. The inmate arrived in medical about 10 minutes later in no visible acute distress other than the look of discomfort I could see on his face. I took his vital signs, which were all within normal range, checked his eyes and pupils, and did a general assessment on him including lung and bowel sounds. At that point I could find nothing abnormal. While doing my assessment, I was asking him questions about his symptoms to try and rule out any medical condition other than a general headache. The only other symptom he said he was experiencing was blurry vision, which can occur with headaches, especially migraines. I checked his visual acuity with the eye chart, but found no major deficit. He said he did not normally wear glasses, so I assumed that the headache was not related to him having blurry vision from being without proper eyewear.

But something was telling me that there was more going on with this man than a simple headache. After probing further into any other symptoms, and finding none, I asked if I could take a fingerstick blood sugar reading, explaining what it was for. The result was shocking. The glucometer didn't have a reading that high! I explained to him what this reading meant, and asked him if he had ever had his blood sugar checked previously, or was told that he was diabetic, and he stated he had not. When asked if diabetes ran in his family, he confirmed that both of his parents were diabetic. Armed with the glucose reading and family history, I asked about unquenchable thirst, hunger, frequent urination, and other indicators of hyperglycemia. When he responded affirmatively to all these questions, I lightheartedly responded that "I thought you told me that you weren't having any other symptoms?" This brought a chuckle and helped ease the anxiety I could see that he was feeling. At that point, I explained to him that all of the symptoms he stated he was experiencing were signs of diabetes, and explained why he had those particular symptoms. He acknowledged understanding everything I was explaining to him.

Luckily the nurse practitioner had not left for the day, so I was able to have him seen immediately. Once evaluated by the NP, treatment orders were written and I administered insulin for the hyperglycemia and ibuprophen for the headache. I also scheduled him for ongoing insulin and blood glucose monitoring. Finally, we started diabetes education with literature and dietary information. Before he left the medical unit, I rechecked his blood sugar to be sure it was in a better range.

Before sending this patient back to his cell, I acknowledged his anxiety and confirmed that we would help him manage this new condition. He seemed much more relaxed after I took the extra time to assure him that he was not going to have to go through this alone.

The Lesson

This story is a reminder to take those few extra minutes to dig deeper when your instinct is telling you that something is wrong. Had I not done this, it's very possible that he may have gone into ketoacidosis during the night and no one would have known until it was too late. Since this experience I am more inclined to check someone's blood sugar than I would have before.

Also, I learned that understanding the patient is so important. For example, this inmate did not normally complain or come to medical frequently with various issues. Yet, this issue was important enough to him to seek out attention. This added to my suspicion that something was not right and to dig further.

Nurse Radar

David Turner, RN, works in a maximum security receiving facility with an average daily population of 1,600 male inmates. Here is his correctional nursing tale.

The Background

I spent the first 20+ years of my nursing career in the Emergency Department (ED) - a role I loved and thought I would never want to leave. Well, time marches on, we get a little older and not as enthusiastic about 12-hour shifts wearing running shoes. After just over 3 years in corrections nursing, I know now that the ED was really just a fancy, fast-paced training ground for nursing in prison. Many of the same personalities, the same demanding behaviors, the same exaggerated complaints, and the same impatience for treatment of a week-old complaint exist behind bars. And, oh yes, the same truly sick or injured patients who had nowhere else to go for care are here, too.

One of the most useful skills I've developed in the ED and utilize now in corrections is *nursing intuition.* I call it *"nursing radar".* You know what I mean, that persistent feeling that "something's not right here." When objective findings are few, lab values normal, x-rays unimpressive, but the little hairs on the back of your neck keep telling you that this person is sick, maybe *really* sick – that's "nurse radar" in action.

The Tale

A short time ago my "nursing radar" kicked in when I assessed a medical emergency for a headache. My patient complained of a frontal headache x4 days and had been seen twice by providers in the last 3 days. NSAID pain relief had failed and the patient complained that the pain was getting worse. Assessment findings were unremarkable, he denied associated nausea/vomiting, tinnitus, vision changes, neck pain, and fever. But that "nursing radar" of mine kept going off. He looked like someone in a lot of pain.

Speaking by phone with the on-call provider, we performed several neuro tests, attempted to read the Snellen chart (the patient has 20/200 vision but could not wear his glasses due to the headache pain) and tested a few gait and stability maneuvers. All with negative results. When I received orders from the on-call provider for NSAID's and a follow-up the next day, I described my feelings of uneasiness. Fortunately, the provider trusted my instincts and agreed to send him out to the local hospital for further evaluation.

We later learned that the patient underwent a CT scan, lab work and a lumbar puncture with CSF evaluation. Much to our surprise, blood work indicated previously undiagnosed HIV infection and the patient's CSF was positive for Cryptococcal Meningitis. He remains in the hospital after over three weeks, receiving both oral and IV antibiotics and amphotericin b infusions. We also learned that Cryptococcal Meningitis is the leading cause of death among people with HIV who do not exhibit signs and symptoms of AIDS. Unfortunately outcomes, with and without treatment, are not encouraging.

The Lesson

Trust your instincts. Trust your judgment. Trust your skills. Trust your "nursing radar". Even if all the objective data seems normal, discuss your concerns with the provider and get the patient to the next level of care. In this situation, higher level diagnostics were needed to find the cause of the headache.

It's Not Always Detox!

Danielle Carbon, LPN, works in a county jail with an average daily census of 1,300. Here is her correctional nursing tale.

The Background

I've been working as a correctional nurse in a county jail for 8 years. One phrase that seems to come out of my mouth time and time again is "It's not always detox." I have learned that even though the signs and symptoms of any condition could be right there slapping you in the face, there could always be something hiding in the shadows.

The Tale

A few years ago I had the privilege of working as infirmary dayshift charge nurse. During report, the off-going charge nurse told me of a patient with a history of drug abuse. Due to the amount he used he was automatically housed in the infirmary and treated for detox. He was approximately three days into the withdrawal protocol, but not showing much improvement.

When I assessed him he was lying in bed - a slender white male in his mid-40's. As he sat up I could see he was weak with fine motor tremors. He denied any specific symptoms, but said he felt sick. A little over a week ago he was diagnosed with tonsillitis and never fully felt better. He reported feeling worse the last two days. His blood pressure was mildly elevated and his pulse was in the 140's. I made a call to the doctor immediately. His diagnosis after we drew stat labs was acute Hashimotos thyroiditis. With treatment he was like a new man. He left the jail being diagnosed and treated for an illness he had no idea he had; and he was fully detoxed from a drug that took over

20 years of his life.

The Lesson

One thing I have learned working corrections is sometimes there will be a zebra in your herd of horses. You always need to keep your eyes open in case one comes your way. Also don't always assume "it's just detox" when a patient with a drug history is looking and feeling ill, because sometimes IT'S NOT!

That Chest Pain Thing

Laura Mish, RN, works in a medium security prison with an average daily population of 3,300 male inmates. Here is one of her correctional nursing tales.

The Background

Having been a correctional nurse at a state prison for nearly 16 years, I have many stories to tell. Some are sad, some are funny, and then there are those that you will never forget. They change your perspective, not only on correctional nursing, but on nursing in general. I have learned invaluable lessons from many of my inmate patients. Here is another one you might like.

The Tale

I was working evening shift one day as the compound nurse, and was called to medical in one of the buildings in general population for an emergency sick call. I was told that there was an inmate coming to medical with chest pain. He arrived shortly thereafter and I began to get information from him about his pain. I noted that he was only in his early 30's. He told me that he was experiencing a feeling of pressure in the middle of his chest that had started earlier in the day. He said that the pain was getting worse as the day went on, but he denied any other symptoms, including pain radiating down his arm or shortness of breath. While assessing him I noted that he was not diaphoretic, and did not seem to be in acute distress. His blood pressure was slightly elevated, but nothing of urgency. At the time I was considering a cardiac issue, but considering he had no other symptoms, I also thought he could be experiencing atypical chest pain. I had asked him if he ever had this type of pain in the past, and he stated that he had not. I thought that possibly he could have a muscle strain since he did tell me that the previous day he had been in the gym area working out.

In an instance such as this, it is very easy to dismiss the issue as muscle strain since he had been exercising, but something told me to do an EKG anyway. The EKG started to print out, and when I saw the results I was SO glad that I had decided to do the EKG. At that moment this inmate was in the process of having an acute MI! I looked over at him and saw that he was suddenly becoming very diaphoretic. I called the LPN to come and sit with him, and I told him "I'll be right back" and practically ran out of the room! While I was calling 911 I asked the LPN to give him aspirin and nitroglycerin, and to recheck his blood pressure. I went back in to him and apologized for my abrupt exit from the room, and told him what was happening. Within a short period of time the paramedics arrived and their EKG also showed an acute MI, so he was quickly transported to the local ER.

About 2 weeks later I was working in our Extended Care Unit when I saw him. He had been housed in there after returning from the hospital. He immediately recognized me, and thanked me for acting so quickly in getting him out of there and to the hospital. He told me that he had to have an angioplasty done immediately after arriving in the ER that day, and said that the doctor in the ER told him that if too much more time had passed before he got to the hospital, his situation would have been very bleak. Turns out he had a major artery that was almost completely blocked! He returned to general population after his stay in the Extended Care Unit and had no further problems.

The Lesson

I often think about this situation, and remind myself to look further into symptoms that an inmate is experiencing. I could have very easily dismissed his chest pain as a muscle strain, but I'm so glad I went a step further and did an EKG. I hope that my story will one day be of help to someone, and be an example of how immediate medical attention and taking that extra step can save someone's life!

References and Resources

The following sources were consulted for fact accuracy in this book. Citation within the text was avoided to improve readability. Learn more about many of the topics in this book by obtaining these documents or online sources. Find other Quick Start resources at correctionalnurse.net/quickstart.

American Nurses Association (2013). *Correctional nursing scope and standards of practice* (2nd ed.). Silver Springs Maryland: American Nurses Association.

American Nurses Association (2015). *Code of ethics for nurses with interpretive statements.* Silver Springs, MD: American Nurses Association. Retrieved from http://www.nursingworld.org/MainMenuCategories/EthicsSta ndards/CodeofEthicsforNurses/Code-of-Ethics-For-Nurses.html

Burns, K. (2010, October 27). *21 ways to avoid job interview anxiety.* Retrieved January 25, 2016, from http://money.usnews.com/money/blogs/outside-voices-careers/2010/10/27/21-ways-to-avoid-job-interview-anxiety

Finding the Meaning in Your Work (n.d.). Retrieved January 21, 2016, from http://www.psychologytoday.com/blog/career-transitions/201402/finding-the-meaning-in-your-work

Flanagan, N. A., & Flanagan, T. J. (2001). Correctional nurses' perceptions of their role, training requirements, and prisoner health care needs. *Journal of Correctional Health Care, 8*(1), 67–85. http://doi.org/10.1177/107834580100800105

Fowler, M. D. M. (Ed.). (2015). *Guide to the code of ethics for nurses: Interpretation and application.* Silver Springs, MD: American Nurses Association.

Kennedy, B., Curtis, K., & Waters, D. (2014). Is there a relationship between personality and choice of nursing specialty: an integrative literature review. *BMC Nursing, 13*(1), 40. http://doi.org/10.1186/s12912-014-0040-z

Knox, C. M. (2013). Dental conditions. In L. Schoenly & C. M. Knox (Eds.), *Essentials of correctional nursing* (pp. 123–140). New York, NY: Springer.

Kripalani, S., Bengtzen, R., Henderson, L. E., & Jacobson, T. A. (2008). Clinical research in low-literacy populations: using teach-back to assess comprehension of informed consent and privacy information. *IRB: Ethics and Human Research, 30*(2), 13–19.

Lewandowski, G. W. (2012). *Is a bad mood contagious?* Retrieved January 25, 2016, from http://www.scientificamerican.com/article/is-a-bad-mood-contagious/

Maroney, M. K. (2005). Caring and custody: Two faces of the same reality. *Journal of Correctional Health Care, 11*(2), 157–169. http://doi.org/10.1177/107834580401100204

McCrae, R. R., & John, O. P. (1992). An introduction to the five-factor model and its applications. *Journal of Personality, 60*(2), 175–215.

National Commission on Correctional Health Care (U.S.) (2014). *Standards for health services in prisons, 2014.* Chicago, IL: National Commission on Correctional Health Care.

Schoenly, L. (2013). Context of correctional nursing. In L. Schoenly & C. M. Knox (Eds.), *Essentials of correctional nursing* (pp. 1–18). New York, NY: Springer.

Schoenly, L. (2014). *Correctional health care patient safety handbook.* Nashville, TN: Enchanted Mountain Press.

Smith, J. (2013). *14 tips for staying calm during a job interview.* Retrieved January 26, 2016, from http://www.forbes.com/sites/jacquelynsmith/2013/03/26/14-tips-for-staying-calm-during-a-job-interview/

Williams, B. A., Stern, M. F., Mellow, J., Safer, M., & Greifinger, R. B. (2012). Aging in correctional custody: setting a policy agenda for older prisoner health care. *American Journal of Public Health, 102*(8), 1475–1481.

Wrzesniewski, A., McCauley, C. R., Rozin, P., & Schwartz, B. (1997). Jobs, careers, and callings: People's relations to their work. Journal of Research in Personality, 31, 21-33

Wrzesniewski, A., Berg, J. M., & Dutton, J. E. (2010, June 1). Managing Yourself: Turn the Job You Have into the Job You Want. Retrieved January 25, 2016, from https://hbr.org/2010/06/managing-yourself-turn-the-job-you-have-into-the-job-you-want

About the Author

Lorry Schoenly is a nurse author and educator specializing in correctional health care. She provides consulting services to jails and prisons across the US, helping to improve professional nursing practice and patient safety. Dr. Schoenly actively promotes correctional health care 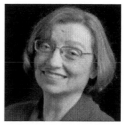 through social media outlets and increases the visibility of the specialty through her popular blog – CorrectionalNurse.Net. Her podcast, Correctional Nursing Today, reviews correctional health care news and interviews correctional health care leaders. She is the recipient of the National Commission on Correctional Health Care 2013 B. Jaye Anno Award of Excellence in Communication. Lorry is author of *The Correctional Health Care Patient Safety Handbook* and co-editor and chapter author of *Essentials of Correctional Nursing*, the first primary practice text for the correctional nursing specialty. She resides in the mountains of north central Pennsylvania.

Made in the USA
San Bernardino, CA
07 October 2016